Alzheimer's Diet Cookbook for Beginners

Nutrient-Rich Recipes for Improved Brain Function, Reduced Inflammation, Better Blood Sugar Control, Weight Management, Increased Energy Levels, and Enhanced Mood

Judy Kelly

Copyright © Judy Kelly, 2024.

All rights reserved. No part of this publication may be reproduced, distributed, or transmitted in any form or by any means, including photocopying, recording, or other electronic or mechanical methods, without the prior written permission of the publisher, except in the case of brief quotations embodied in critical reviews and certain other noncommercial uses permitted by copyright law.

Table of Content

Introduction.. 4

Understanding Alzheimer's Disease........................... 5

   Importance of Diet in Alzheimer's Management............ 6

Chapter 1: The Alzheimer's Diet Basics...................... 8

   Overview of the Alzheimer's Diet.................................. 8

   - Key Nutrients for Brain Health..................................... 8

   - Foods to Avoid... 10

Chapter 2: Breakfast Recipes..................................... 12

Chapter 3: Lunch Recipes.. 30

Chapter 4: Dinner Recipes... 50

Chapter 5: Snacks and Desserts............................... 72

Chapter 6: Caregiver Support.................................... 78

   Tips for Caregivers.. 79

   Self-Care for Caregivers.. 80

Chapter 7: 28-Day Meal Plan...................................... 82

Conclusion... 88

Introduction

Welcome to the "Alzheimer's Diet Cookbook for Beginners." This cookbook is more than just a collection of recipes; it's a guide to nurturing the mind and body through the power of food. Alzheimer's disease is a challenging journey, both for those diagnosed and their loved ones. While there is no cure, there are ways to support brain health and overall well-being, and one of the most impactful ways is through diet.

For many, the idea of changing their diet can be daunting. It may conjure images of bland meals and restrictive eating. However, this cookbook is here to show you that eating for brain health can be delicious, satisfying, and even joyful. It's about embracing the vibrant colors and flavors of wholesome ingredients and understanding the profound impact they can have on our bodies and minds.

Each recipe in this cookbook is carefully crafted to not only taste good but also to nourish your brain and body. From brain-boosting breakfasts to comforting dinners, every dish is designed with your well-being in mind. The recipes feature ingredients rich in antioxidants, vitamins, and minerals that support cognitive function, reduce inflammation, regulate blood sugar, and promote overall health.

But this cookbook is not just about what you eat; it's also about how you eat. It includes a 28-day meal plan, meal planner journal, and shopping list templates to help you seamlessly integrate these recipes into your life. It's about creating a sustainable and enjoyable way of eating that supports your health and happiness.

Whether you're cooking for yourself, a family member, or a friend with Alzheimer's disease, know that every meal you prepare is an act of love and care. Together, let's nourish our bodies and minds, one delicious recipe at a time.

Understanding Alzheimer's Disease

Alzheimer's disease is a progressive neurodegenerative disorder that affects millions of people worldwide. It is the most common cause of dementia, a term used to describe a decline in cognitive function severe enough to interfere with daily life. Alzheimer's disease primarily affects older adults, with the risk increasing with age. While the exact cause of Alzheimer's disease is not fully understood, it is believed to be a combination of genetic, environmental, and lifestyle factors.

One of the hallmarks of Alzheimer's disease is the accumulation of abnormal protein deposits in the brain, known as plaques and tangles. These deposits interfere with the communication between nerve cells and ultimately lead to cell death and tissue loss in the brain. As a result, individuals with Alzheimer's disease experience a gradual decline in memory, thinking, and reasoning skills.

In addition to cognitive symptoms, Alzheimer's disease can also cause changes in behavior and personality. People with Alzheimer's may become confused, agitated, or withdrawn. They may also have difficulty with language and communication, as well as with recognizing familiar people and objects.

Currently, there is no cure for Alzheimer's disease. However, there are treatments available that can help manage symptoms and improve quality of life for some individuals. These treatments include medications that can temporarily improve cognitive function or manage behavioral symptoms.

While Alzheimer's disease is a devastating condition, there is hope. Research into the causes and treatments for Alzheimer's is ongoing, and advances are being made every day. By raising awareness, supporting research, and providing compassionate care for those affected by Alzheimer's, we can work together to make a difference in the fight against this disease.

Importance of Diet in Alzheimer's Management

The importance of diet in Alzheimer's management cannot be overstated. While diet alone cannot cure or prevent Alzheimer's disease, it plays a crucial role in supporting overall brain health and may help slow the progression of the disease. Here are several key reasons why diet is important in Alzheimer's management:

1. Nutrient Intake: A diet rich in nutrients, such as antioxidants, vitamins, and minerals, can support brain health and function. These nutrients help protect brain cells from damage and promote the growth of new brain cells.

2. Inflammation: Chronic inflammation is believed to play a role in the development and progression of Alzheimer's disease. A diet high in anti-inflammatory foods, such as fruits, vegetables, whole grains, and healthy fats, can help reduce inflammation in the brain and throughout the body.

3. Blood Sugar Control: Studies have shown that high blood sugar levels may increase the risk of developing Alzheimer's disease. Eating a diet low in refined sugars and high in complex carbohydrates can help regulate blood sugar levels and reduce the risk of insulin resistance, a condition that can lead to diabetes and increase the risk of Alzheimer's.

4. Heart Health: There is a strong connection between heart health and brain health. A diet that is good for the heart, such as one low in saturated fats and cholesterol, can also be beneficial for the brain. This type of diet can help reduce the risk of cardiovascular disease, which is a risk factor for Alzheimer's.

5. Weight Management: Maintaining a healthy weight is important for overall health and can help reduce the risk of developing Alzheimer's disease. A diet that is balanced and nutritious can help support weight management and reduce the risk of obesity, which is a risk factor for Alzheimer's.

6. Mood and Behavior: Diet can also have an impact on mood and behavior, which can be important considerations for individuals with Alzheimer's disease. Eating a diet that is rich in omega-3 fatty acids, for example, may help improve mood and reduce the risk of depression, which is common in people with Alzheimer's.

Overall, a healthy diet can play a significant role in Alzheimer's management by supporting brain health, reducing inflammation, regulating blood sugar, supporting heart health, and managing weight. While diet is just one piece of the puzzle in Alzheimer's management, it is an important piece that should not be overlooked.

Chapter 1: The Alzheimer's Diet Basics

Overview of the Alzheimer's Diet

The "Alzheimer's Diet," also known as the MIND diet (Mediterranean-DASH Intervention for Neurodegenerative Delay), is a dietary pattern that emphasizes foods that are believed to support brain health and reduce the risk of Alzheimer's disease. It combines elements of the Mediterranean diet and the DASH (Dietary Approaches to Stop Hypertension) diet, both of which have been associated with numerous health benefits, including improved brain function.

The Alzheimer's Diet is rich in fruits, vegetables, whole grains, lean proteins, and healthy fats, while limiting processed foods, red meat, and sweets. It includes foods that are high in antioxidants, such as berries, nuts, and leafy greens, which are thought to protect the brain from oxidative stress and inflammation. The diet also includes foods rich in omega-3 fatty acids, such as fish, which are believed to support brain health and cognitive function.

Several studies have suggested that following a diet similar to the Alzheimer's Diet may help reduce the risk of developing Alzheimer's disease and slow the progression of the disease in those who already have it. While more research is needed to fully understand the impact of diet on Alzheimer's disease, adopting a healthy dietary pattern like the Alzheimer's Diet may offer numerous benefits for brain health and overall well-being.

- Key Nutrients for Brain Health

Several nutrients are essential for brain health and may play a role in reducing the risk of Alzheimer's disease and supporting cognitive function. Some of the key nutrients include:

1. Omega-3 fatty acids: Found in fatty fish like salmon, trout, and sardines, as well as in flaxseeds, chia seeds, and walnuts, omega-3 fatty acids are

important for brain health. They help build cell membranes in the brain and have anti-inflammatory effects, which may protect against Alzheimer's disease.

2. Antioxidants: Antioxidants help protect the brain from oxidative stress, which can damage cells and contribute to cognitive decline. Foods rich in antioxidants include berries (such as blueberries, strawberries, and raspberries), dark chocolate, and colorful fruits and vegetables like spinach, kale, and beets.

3. Vitamin E: Vitamin E is an antioxidant that may help protect neurons or nerve cells. Foods high in vitamin E include nuts, seeds, spinach, and broccoli.

4. Vitamin B12: Vitamin B12 plays a role in the production of brain chemicals and the maintenance of myelin, which insulates nerve fibers. It is found in animal products like meat, fish, eggs, and dairy products.

5. Vitamin D: Vitamin D is important for brain health and may help reduce the risk of cognitive decline. It is found in fatty fish, fortified dairy products, and exposure to sunlight.

6. Magnesium: Magnesium is involved in hundreds of biochemical reactions in the body, including those that support brain function. It is found in nuts, seeds, whole grains, and leafy green vegetables.

7. Flavonoids: Flavonoids are a group of antioxidants found in plant foods that may help improve memory and cognitive function. Foods rich in flavonoids include berries, citrus fruits, apples, onions, and tea.

Including these nutrients in your diet can help support brain health and may reduce the risk of Alzheimer's disease. A diet rich in fruits, vegetables, whole grains, lean proteins, and healthy fats can provide these nutrients and support overall brain health.

- Foods to Avoid

While there is no single "Alzheimer's diet" that guarantees prevention or cure, certain foods are best avoided or limited to support brain health and reduce the risk of cognitive decline. These include:

1. Trans fats: Found in fried foods, baked goods, and processed snacks, trans fats can increase inflammation and may contribute to the development of cognitive impairment.

2. Saturated fats: High intake of saturated fats, found in red meat, butter, and full-fat dairy products, has been associated with an increased risk of Alzheimer's disease and cognitive decline.

3. Added sugars: Foods and beverages high in added sugars, such as soda, candy, and desserts, can lead to inflammation and insulin resistance, which are harmful to brain health.

4. Processed foods: Processed foods like fast food, chips, and convenience meals often contain high levels of unhealthy fats, sugars, and sodium, which can negatively impact brain health.

5. Highly processed carbohydrates: Refined grains like white bread, white rice, and pasta can lead to spikes in blood sugar levels, which may contribute to inflammation and cognitive decline.

6. Excessive alcohol: While moderate alcohol consumption may have some health benefits, excessive alcohol intake can damage brain cells and increase the risk of cognitive impairment.

7. Highly salted foods: Consuming too much salt can lead to high blood pressure, which is a risk factor for cognitive decline and Alzheimer's disease.

It's important to note that while these foods should be limited, a balanced diet that includes a variety of nutrient-rich foods is key to supporting overall health and brain function.

Chapter 2: Breakfast Recipes

1. BLUEBERRY OATMEAL

Ingredients:
- 1/2 cup rolled oats
- 1 cup water or milk of choice
- 1/2 cup blueberries
- 1 tablespoon honey or maple syrup (optional)
- 1/2 teaspoon cinnamon

Instructions:
1. In a small saucepan, combine oats and water or milk. Bring to a boil, then reduce heat and simmer for 5 minutes.
2. Stir in blueberries, honey or maple syrup (if using), and cinnamon. Cook for an additional 2-3 minutes.
3. Remove from heat and let cool slightly before serving.

Nutritional Info: (per serving)
- Calories: 250
- Protein: 7g
- Fat: 3g
- Carbohydrates: 50g
- Fiber: 8g

Prep Time: 2 minutes
Cook Time: 8 minutes
Serving: 1

---

2. AVOCADO TOAST

Ingredients:
- 1 slice whole grain bread

- 1/2 avocado
- Salt and pepper to taste
- Optional toppings: sliced tomatoes, red pepper flakes, or a drizzle of balsamic glaze

Instructions:
1. Toast the bread until golden brown.
2. Mash the avocado and spread it evenly on the toast.
3. Season with salt and pepper, and add any additional toppings as desired.

Nutritional Info: (per serving)
- Calories: 200
- Protein: 5g
- Fat: 10g
- Carbohydrates: 25g
- Fiber: 7g

Prep Time: 5 minutes
Cook Time: 2 minutes
Serving: 1

---

3. CHIA SEED PUDDING

Ingredients:
- 2 tablespoons chia seeds
- 1/2 cup almond milk (or any milk of choice)
- 1/2 teaspoon vanilla extract
- 1 tablespoon maple syrup (optional)
- Fresh fruit for topping

Instructions:
1. In a bowl, mix chia seeds, almond milk, vanilla extract, and maple syrup (if using). Stir well.

2. Cover and refrigerate overnight, or for at least 2 hours, until the mixture thickens.
3. Serve topped with fresh fruit.

Nutritional Info: (per serving)
- Calories: 150
- Protein: 4g
- Fat: 8g
- Carbohydrates: 15g
- Fiber: 7g

Prep Time: 5 minutes
Cook Time: 0 minutes
Serving: 1

---

4. BANANA PANCAKES

Ingredients:
- 1 ripe banana
- 2 eggs
- 1/4 teaspoon baking powder (optional)
- Butter or oil for cooking
- Optional toppings: maple syrup, berries, or nuts

Instructions:
1. In a bowl, mash the banana until smooth. Add eggs and baking powder, and mix well.
2. Heat a skillet over medium heat and add butter or oil.
3. Pour small amounts of the batter onto the skillet to form pancakes. Cook for 2-3 minutes per side, until golden brown.
4. Serve with your choice of toppings.

Nutritional Info: (per serving, without toppings)

- Calories: 250
- Protein: 12g
- Fat: 10g
- Carbohydrates: 30g
- Fiber: 3g

Prep Time: 5 minutes
Cook Time: 5 minutes
Serving: 1-2

---

5. GREEK YOGURT PARFAIT

Ingredients:
- 1/2 cup Greek yogurt
- 1/4 cup granola
- 1/2 cup mixed berries
- Honey or maple syrup for drizzling (optional)

Instructions:
1. In a glass or bowl, layer Greek yogurt, granola, and mixed berries.
2. Repeat layers until ingredients are used up.
3. Drizzle with honey or maple syrup if desired.

Nutritional Info: (per serving)
- Calories: 250
- Protein: 15g
- Fat: 5g
- Carbohydrates: 35g
- Fiber: 5g

Prep Time: 5 minutes
Cook Time: 0 minutes
Serving: 1

6. SPINACH AND FETA OMELET

Ingredients:
- 2 eggs
- 1/4 cup chopped spinach
- 2 tablespoons crumbled feta cheese
- Salt and pepper to taste
- 1 teaspoon olive oil

Instructions:
1. In a bowl, beat the eggs with a fork. Add spinach, feta cheese, salt, and pepper, and mix well.
2. Heat olive oil in a skillet over medium heat. Pour the egg mixture into the skillet.
3. Cook for 2-3 minutes, or until the edges start to set. Using a spatula, gently lift the edges of the omelette and tilt the skillet to let the uncooked egg flow underneath.
4. Continue cooking for another 2-3 minutes, or until the omelet is fully cooked. Fold it in half and serve hot.

Nutritional Info: (per serving)
- Calories: 250
- Protein: 20g
- Fat: 18g
- Carbohydrates: 3g
- Fiber: 1g

Prep Time: 5 minutes
Cook Time: 5 minutes
Serving: 1

---

7. APPLE CINNAMON QUINOA PORRIDGE

Ingredients:
- 1/2 cup quinoa, rinsed
- 1 cup water or milk of choice
- 1 apple, peeled and diced
- 1/2 teaspoon cinnamon
- 1 tablespoon honey or maple syrup (optional)

Instructions:
1. In a saucepan, combine quinoa and water or milk. Bring to a boil, then reduce heat and simmer for 15 minutes, or until quinoa is tender.
2. Stir in diced apple, cinnamon, and honey or maple syrup (if using). Cook for an additional 5 minutes.
3. Remove from heat and let cool slightly before serving.

Nutritional Info: (per serving)
- Calories: 300
- Protein: 8g
- Fat: 3g
- Carbohydrates: 60g
- Fiber: 7g

Prep Time: 5 minutes
Cook Time: 20 minutes
Serving: 1

---

8. PEANUT BUTTER BANANA SMOOTHIE

Ingredients:
- 1 banana
- 1 tablespoon peanut butter
- 1/2 cup Greek yogurt

- 1/2 cup almond milk (or any milk of choice)
- 1/2 teaspoon honey (optional)
- Ice cubes (optional)

Instructions:
1. Combine all ingredients in a blender and blend until smooth.
2. Add more milk if needed to reach desired consistency.
3. Pour into a glass and serve immediately.

Nutritional Info: (per serving)
- Calories: 300
- Protein: 15g
- Fat: 10g
- Carbohydrates: 40g
- Fiber: 5g

Prep Time: 5 minutes
Cook Time: 0 minutes
Serving: 1

---

9. WHOLE GRAIN BERRY MUFFINS

Ingredients:
- 1 1/2 cups whole wheat flour
- 1/2 cup oats
- 1/2 cup honey or maple syrup
- 1/4 cup coconut oil, melted
- 1/2 cup almond milk
- 2 eggs
- 1 teaspoon baking powder
- 1/2 teaspoon baking soda
- 1/2 teaspoon cinnamon
- 1 cup mixed berries (such as blueberries, raspberries, or strawberries)

Instructions:
1. Preheat the oven to 350°F (175°C) and line a muffin tin with liners.
2. In a large bowl, mix together flour, oats, baking powder, baking soda, and cinnamon.
3. In another bowl, whisk together honey or maple syrup, coconut oil, almond milk, and eggs.
4. Pour wet ingredients into dry ingredients and mix until just combined. Fold in berries.
5. Divide batter evenly among muffin cups and bake for 20-25 minutes, or until a toothpick inserted into the center comes out clean.

Nutritional Info: (per serving)
- Calories: 200
- Protein: 5g
- Fat: 7g
- Carbohydrates: 30g
- Fiber: 4g

Prep Time: 10 minutes
Cook Time: 20-25 minutes
Serving: 12 muffins

---

10. TURMERIC CHICKPEA SCRAMBLE

Ingredients:
- 1 can (15 oz) chickpeas, drained and rinsed
- 1 tablespoon olive oil
- 1/2 onion, chopped
- 1/2 bell pepper, chopped
- 1/2 teaspoon turmeric
- Salt and pepper to taste
- Fresh parsley for garnish

Instructions:
1. In a skillet, heat olive oil over medium heat. Add onion and bell pepper, and sauté until softened.
2. Add chickpeas, turmeric, salt, and pepper. Cook for another 5 minutes, mashing some of the chickpeas with a fork.
3. Serve hot, garnished with fresh parsley.

Nutritional Info: (per serving)
- Calories: 250
- Protein: 10g
- Fat: 7g
- Carbohydrates: 35g
- Fiber: 10g

Prep Time: 10 minutes
Cook Time: 10 minutes
Serving: 2

---

11. OVERNIGHT CHIA SEED PUDDING

Ingredients:
- 1/4 cup chia seeds
- 1 cup almond milk (or any milk of choice)
- 1 tablespoon honey or maple syrup
- 1/2 teaspoon vanilla extract
- Fresh fruit for topping

Instructions:
1. In a bowl, mix chia seeds, almond milk, honey or maple syrup, and vanilla extract. Stir well.
2. Cover and refrigerate overnight, or for at least 2 hours, until the mixture thickens.
3. Serve topped with fresh fruit.

Nutritional Info: (per serving)
- Calories: 200
- Protein: 5g
- Fat: 10g
- Carbohydrates: 25g
- Fiber: 10g

Prep Time: 5 minutes
Cook Time: 0 minutes
Serving: 2

---

12. SWEET POTATO BREAKFAST BOWL

Ingredients:
- 1 medium sweet potato, peeled and cubed
- 1 tablespoon olive oil
- 1/2 teaspoon paprika
- Salt and pepper to taste
- 2 eggs
- 1/4 avocado, sliced
- Fresh cilantro for garnish

Instructions:
1. Preheat the oven to 400°F (200°C).
2. In a bowl, toss sweet potato cubes with olive oil, paprika, salt, and pepper. Spread on a baking sheet and bake for 20-25 minutes, or until tender.
3. Meanwhile, cook eggs to your liking (boiled, scrambled, or fried).
4. In a bowl, layer sweet potatoes, eggs, and avocado slices. Garnish with fresh cilantro.

Nutritional Info: (per serving)
- Calories: 300
- Protein: 12g
- Fat: 15g
- Carbohydrates: 30g
- Fiber: 7g

Prep Time: 10 minutes
Cook Time: 25 minutes
Serving: 1

---

13. BERRY AND ALMOND BUTTER TOAST

Ingredients:
- 1 slice whole grain bread, toasted
- 1 tablespoon almond butter
- 1/2 cup mixed berries
- 1 teaspoon honey or maple syrup (optional)

Instructions:
1. Spread almond butter on the toast.
2. Top with mixed berries.
3. Drizzle with honey or maple syrup if desired.

Nutritional Info: (per serving)
- Calories: 250
- Protein: 8g
- Fat: 10g
- Carbohydrates: 35g
- Fiber: 7g

Prep Time: 5 minutes
Cook Time: 0 minutes

Serving: 1

---

14. SPINACH AND TOMATO EGG MUFFINS

Ingredients:
- 4 eggs
- 1/4 cup milk of choice
- 1 cup chopped spinach
- 1/2 cup diced tomatoes
- Salt and pepper to taste
- 1/4 cup shredded cheese (optional)

Instructions:
1. Preheat the oven to 350°F (175°C) and grease a muffin tin.
2. In a bowl, whisk together eggs, milk, salt, and pepper.
3. Stir in chopped spinach and diced tomatoes.
4. Pour the mixture into the muffin tin, filling each cup about 3/4 full. Sprinkle with shredded cheese if using.
5. Bake for 20-25 minutes, or until the egg muffins are set and lightly golden.

Nutritional Info: (per serving, 2 muffins)
- Calories: 200
- Protein: 14g
- Fat: 10g
- Carbohydrates: 10g
- Fiber: 2g

Prep Time: 10 minutes
Cook Time: 20-25 minutes
Serving: 1

---

15. BANANA CHOCOLATE CHIP SMOOTHIE BOWL

Ingredients:
- 1 frozen banana
- 1/2 cup almond milk (or any milk of choice)
- 1 tablespoon cocoa powder
- 1 tablespoon almond butter
- 1 tablespoon honey or maple syrup (optional)
- 2 tablespoons chocolate chips
- Toppings: sliced banana, granola, chocolate chips

Instructions:
1. In a blender, combine frozen banana, almond milk, cocoa powder, almond butter, and honey or maple syrup. Blend until smooth.
2. Pour into a bowl and top with chocolate chips, sliced banana, and granola.

Nutritional Info: (per serving)
- Calories: 350
- Protein: 5g
- Fat: 15g
- Carbohydrates: 50g
- Fiber: 8g

Prep Time: 5 minutes
Cook Time: 0 minutes
Serving: 1

16. QUINOA FRUIT SALAD

Ingredients:
- 1/2 cup cooked quinoa
- 1/2 cup mixed fresh fruit (such as berries, kiwi, and mango)
- 1 tablespoon chopped nuts (such as almonds or walnuts)
- 1 tablespoon honey or maple syrup

- 1/2 teaspoon cinnamon

Instructions:
1. In a bowl, combine cooked quinoa, mixed fruit, and chopped nuts.
2. Drizzle with honey or maple syrup and sprinkle with cinnamon. Mix well.
3. Serve chilled.

Nutritional Info: (per serving)
- Calories: 250
- Protein: 5g
- Fat: 5g
- Carbohydrates: 50g
- Fiber: 7g

Prep Time: 10 minutes
Cook Time: 15 minutes
Serving: 1

---

17. BREAKFAST BURRITO

Ingredients:
- 1 whole wheat tortilla
- 2 eggs, scrambled
- 1/4 cup black beans, drained and rinsed
- 1/4 cup diced bell peppers
- 1/4 cup shredded cheese
- Salsa and avocado for topping

Instructions:
1. Heat a skillet over medium heat and lightly toast the tortilla.
2. Fill the tortilla with scrambled eggs, black beans, diced bell peppers, and shredded cheese.
3. Roll up the tortilla to form a burrito.

4. Serve with salsa and avocado on top.

Nutritional Info: (per serving)
- Calories: 350
- Protein: 20g
- Fat: 15g
- Carbohydrates: 30g
- Fiber: 8g

Prep Time: 10 minutes
Cook Time: 10 minutes
Serving: 1

---

18. APPLE CINNAMON BAKED OATMEAL

Ingredients:
- 1 cup rolled oats
- 1/2 teaspoon baking powder
- 1 teaspoon cinnamon
- 1/4 teaspoon salt
- 1 cup almond milk (or any milk of choice)
- 1 egg
- 1/4 cup maple syrup
- 1 teaspoon vanilla extract
- 1 apple, peeled and diced
- 1/4 cup chopped nuts (such as walnuts or pecans)

Instructions:
1. Preheat the oven to 350°F (175°C) and grease a baking dish.
2. In a bowl, mix together oats, baking powder, cinnamon, and salt.
3. In another bowl, whisk together almond milk, egg, maple syrup, and vanilla extract.
4. Pour the wet ingredients into the dry ingredients and mix well. Stir in diced apple and chopped nuts.

5. Pour the mixture into the prepared baking dish and bake for 30-35 minutes, or until set and golden brown.

Nutritional Info: (per serving)
- Calories: 300
- Protein: 8g
- Fat: 10g
- Carbohydrates: 45g
- Fiber: 6g

Prep Time: 10 minutes
Cook Time: 30-35 minutes
Serving: 4

---

19. GREEN SMOOTHIE

Ingredients:
- 1 cup spinach
- 1/2 banana
- 1/2 cup frozen mango chunks
- 1/2 cup almond milk (or any milk of choice)
- 1/2 cup Greek yogurt
- 1 tablespoon honey or maple syrup (optional)

Instructions:
1. Combine all ingredients in a blender and blend until smooth.
2. Add more almond milk if needed to reach desired consistency.
3. Pour into a glass and serve immediately.

Nutritional Info: (per serving)
- Calories: 200
- Protein: 10g
- Fat: 3g

- Carbohydrates: 40g
- Fiber: 5g

Prep Time: 5 minutes
Cook Time: 0 minutes
Serving: 1

---

20. BREAKFAST HASH

Ingredients:
- 1 sweet potato, peeled and diced
- 1/2 onion, chopped
- 1 bell pepper, chopped
- 2 tablespoons olive oil
- 1/2 teaspoon paprika
- Salt and pepper to taste
- 2 eggs
- Fresh parsley for garnish

Instructions:
1. Heat olive oil in a skillet over medium heat. Add sweet potato, onion, and bell pepper. Cook until vegetables are tender, about 10-15 minutes.
2. Season with paprika, salt, and pepper.
3. Push the vegetables to the side of the skillet and crack the eggs into the empty space. Cook until the eggs are done to your liking.
4. Serve hot, garnished with fresh parsley.

Nutritional Info: (per serving)
- Calories: 300
- Protein: 10g
- Fat: 15g
- Carbohydrates: 35g
- Fiber: 6g

Prep Time: 10 minutes
Cook Time: 15 minutes
Serving: 2

Chapter 3: Lunch Recipes

1. CHICKEN AND VEGETABLE STIR-FRY

Ingredients:
- 1 tablespoon olive oil
- 1/2 onion, chopped
- 2 garlic cloves, minced
- 1/2 cup sliced carrots
- 1/2 cup broccoli florets
- 1/2 cup sliced bell peppers
- 1/2 cup sliced mushrooms
- 1/2 cup snap peas
- 1 small chicken breast, cooked and sliced
- 2 tablespoons soy sauce
- 1 tablespoon honey
- Cooked brown rice for serving

Instructions:
1. Heat olive oil in a large skillet over medium heat. Add onion and garlic, and sauté for 1 minute.
2. Add carrots, broccoli, bell peppers, mushrooms, and snap peas. Cook, stirring occasionally, until vegetables are tender-crisp.
3. Add sliced chicken breast, soy sauce, and honey. Cook for another 2-3 minutes, stirring gently.
4. Serve over cooked brown rice.

Nutritional Info: (per serving)
- Calories: 400
- Protein: 25g
- Fat: 15g
- Carbohydrates: 40g
- Fiber: 6g

Prep Time: 15 minutes

Cook Time: 15 minutes
Serving: 1

---

2. TUNA SALAD LETTUCE WRAPS

Ingredients:
- 1 can (5 oz) tuna, drained
- 1/4 cup diced celery
- 1/4 cup diced red onion
- 2 tablespoons plain Greek yogurt
- 1 tablespoon lemon juice
- Salt and pepper to taste
- Lettuce leaves for wrapping

Instructions:
1. In a bowl, combine tuna, celery, red onion, Greek yogurt, lemon juice, salt, and pepper.
2. Spoon the tuna salad into lettuce leaves and wrap.

Nutritional Info: (per serving)
- Calories: 200
- Protein: 20g
- Fat: 5g
- Carbohydrates: 10g
- Fiber: 3g

Prep Time: 10 minutes
Cook Time: 0 minutes
Serving: 2

---

3. CHICKEN AND VEGETABLE SOUP

Ingredients:
- 1 tablespoon olive oil
- 1/2 onion, chopped
- 2 garlic cloves, minced
- 1 carrot, diced
- 1 celery stalk, diced
- 4 cups chicken broth
- 1 cup diced cooked chicken breast
- 1/2 cup frozen peas
- Salt and pepper to taste
- Fresh parsley for garnish

Instructions:
1. Heat olive oil in a large pot over medium heat. Add onion and garlic, and sauté until softened.
2. Add carrot and celery, and cook for another 5 minutes.
3. Pour in chicken broth and bring to a simmer.
4. Add chicken breast and frozen peas. Cook for another 5 minutes, or until heated through.
5. Season with salt and pepper. Garnish with fresh parsley before serving.

Nutritional Info: (per serving)
- Calories: 250
- Protein: 20g
- Fat: 10g
- Carbohydrates: 20g
- Fiber: 4g

Prep Time: 10 minutes
Cook Time: 20 minutes
Serving: 4

---

4. SALMON AND VEGETABLE STIR-FRY

Ingredients:
- 1 tablespoon olive oil
- 1 garlic clove, minced
- 1 teaspoon grated ginger
- 1/2 cup sliced carrots
- 1/2 cup broccoli florets
- 1/2 cup sliced bell peppers
- 1/2 cup sliced mushrooms
- 1/2 cup snap peas
- 1 small salmon filet, cooked and flaked
- 2 tablespoons soy sauce
- 1 tablespoon honey
- Cooked brown rice for serving

Instructions:
1. Heat olive oil in a large skillet over medium heat. Add garlic and ginger, and sauté for 1 minute.
2. Add carrots, broccoli, bell peppers, mushrooms, and snap peas. Cook, stirring occasionally, until vegetables are tender-crisp.
3. Add flaked salmon, soy sauce, and honey. Cook for another 2-3 minutes, stirring gently.
4. Serve over cooked brown rice.

Nutritional Info: (per serving)
- Calories: 400
- Protein: 25g
- Fat: 15g
- Carbohydrates: 40g
- Fiber: 6g

Prep Time: 15 minutes
Cook Time: 15 minutes
Serving: 1

5. TURKEY AND AVOCADO WRAPS

Ingredients:
- 1 large whole wheat tortilla
- 2 tablespoons hummus
- 2 slices turkey breast
- 1/4 avocado, sliced
- 1/4 cup mixed greens

Instructions:
1. Spread hummus evenly over the tortilla.
2. Layer turkey breast, avocado slices, and mixed greens on top.
3. Roll up the tortilla tightly, and cut into slices if desired.

Nutritional Info: (per serving)
- Calories: 300
- Protein: 20g
- Fat: 10g
- Carbohydrates: 30g
- Fiber: 7g

Prep Time: 5 minutes
Cook Time: 0 minutes
Serving: 1

---

6. MEDITERRANEAN CHICKPEA SALAD

Ingredients:
- 1 can (15 oz) chickpeas, drained and rinsed
- 1/2 cucumber, diced
- 1/2 cup cherry tomatoes, halved
- 1/4 cup diced red onion
- 1/4 cup chopped fresh parsley

- Juice of 1 lemon
- 2 tablespoons olive oil
- Salt and pepper to taste
- Crumbled feta cheese (optional)

Instructions:
1. In a large bowl, combine chickpeas, cucumber, cherry tomatoes, red onion, and parsley.
2. In a small bowl, whisk together lemon juice, olive oil, salt, and pepper.
3. Pour the dressing over the salad and toss to coat.
4. Sprinkle with crumbled feta cheese if desired.

Nutritional Info: (per serving)
- Calories: 350
- Protein: 15g
- Fat: 15g
- Carbohydrates: 40g
- Fiber: 10g

Prep Time: 10 minutes
Cook Time: 0 minutes
Serving: 2

---

7. CHICKEN AND VEGETABLE SOUP

Ingredients:
- 1 tablespoon olive oil
- 1/2 onion, chopped
- 2 garlic cloves, minced
- 1 carrot, diced
- 1 celery stalk, diced
- 4 cups chicken broth
- 1 cup diced cooked chicken breast

- 1/2 cup frozen peas
- Salt and pepper to taste
- Fresh parsley for garnish

Instructions:
1. Heat olive oil in a large pot over medium heat. Add onion and garlic, and sauté until softened.
2. Add carrot and celery, and cook for another 5 minutes.
3. Pour in chicken broth and bring to a simmer.
4. Add chicken breast and frozen peas. Cook for another 5 minutes, or until heated through.
5. Season with salt and pepper. Garnish with fresh parsley before serving.

Nutritional Info: (per serving)
- Calories: 250
- Protein: 20g
- Fat: 10g
- Carbohydrates: 20g
- Fiber: 4g

Prep Time: 10 minutes
Cook Time: 20 minutes
Serving: 4

---

8. TUNA SALAD STUFFED AVOCADOS

Ingredients:
- 2 avocados, halved and pitted
- 1 can (5 oz) tuna, drained
- 1/4 cup diced red onion
- 1/4 cup diced celery
- 1/4 cup plain Greek yogurt
- 1 tablespoon lemon juice

- Salt and pepper to taste
- Mixed greens for serving

Instructions:
1. In a bowl, combine tuna, red onion, celery, Greek yogurt, lemon juice, salt, and pepper.
2. Spoon the tuna salad into the avocado halves.
3. Serve on a bed of mixed greens.

Nutritional Info: (per serving)
- Calories: 300
- Protein: 20g
- Fat: 20g
- Carbohydrates: 15g
- Fiber: 10g

Prep Time: 10 minutes
Cook Time: 0 minutes
Serving: 2

---

9. GREEK QUINOA SALAD

Ingredients:
- 1 cup cooked quinoa
- 1/2 cucumber, diced
- 1/2 cup cherry tomatoes, halved
- 1/4 cup diced red onion
- 1/4 cup chopped fresh parsley
- 1/4 cup crumbled feta cheese
- Juice of 1 lemon
- 2 tablespoons olive oil
- Salt and pepper to taste

Instructions:
1. In a large bowl, combine quinoa, cucumber, cherry tomatoes, red onion, parsley, and feta cheese.
2. In a small bowl, whisk together lemon juice, olive oil, salt, and pepper.
3. Pour the dressing over the salad and toss to combine.

Nutritional Info: (per serving)
- Calories: 350
- Protein: 10g
- Fat: 20g
- Carbohydrates: 30g
- Fiber: 5g

Prep Time: 10 minutes
Cook Time: 0 minutes
Serving: 2

---

10. SWEET POTATO AND BLACK BEAN QUESADILLAS

Ingredients:
- 1 large sweet potato, peeled and diced
- 1 can (15 oz) black beans, drained and rinsed
- 1 teaspoon cumin
- 1/2 teaspoon chili powder
- Salt and pepper to taste
- 4 whole wheat tortillas
- 1 cup shredded cheese (such as cheddar or Monterey Jack)
- Salsa and Greek yogurt for serving

Instructions:
1. Steam or microwave the sweet potato until tender. Mash with a fork.
2. In a bowl, combine mashed sweet potato, black beans, cumin, chili powder, salt, and pepper.

3. Divide the mixture evenly among 2 tortillas. Top each with 1/2 cup shredded cheese and another tortilla.
4. Heat a large skillet over medium heat. Cook each quesadilla for 3-4 minutes per side, or until the cheese is melted and the tortillas are crispy.
5. Cut into wedges and serve with salsa and Greek yogurt.

Nutritional Info: (per serving)
- Calories: 400
- Protein: 20g
- Fat: 15g
- Carbohydrates: 50g
- Fiber: 10g

Prep Time: 15 minutes
Cook Time: 15 minutes
Serving: 2

---

11. CHICKEN AND VEGETABLE STIR-FRY

Ingredients:
- 1 tablespoon olive oil
- 1 garlic clove, minced
- 1 teaspoon grated ginger
- 1/2 cup sliced carrots
- 1/2 cup broccoli florets
- 1/2 cup sliced bell peppers
- 1/2 cup sliced mushrooms
- 1/2 cup snap peas
- 1 small chicken breast, cooked and sliced
- 2 tablespoons soy sauce
- 1 tablespoon honey
- Cooked brown rice for serving

Instructions:
1. Heat olive oil in a large skillet over medium heat. Add garlic and ginger, and sauté for 1 minute.
2. Add carrots, broccoli, bell peppers, mushrooms, and snap peas. Cook, stirring occasionally, until vegetables are tender-crisp.
3. Add sliced chicken breast, soy sauce, and honey. Cook for another 2-3 minutes, stirring gently.
4. Serve over cooked brown rice.

Nutritional Info: (per serving)
- Calories: 400
- Protein: 25g
- Fat: 15g
- Carbohydrates: 40g
- Fiber: 6g

Prep Time: 15 minutes
Cook Time: 15 minutes
Serving: 1

---

12. TUNA SALAD LETTUCE WRAPS

Ingredients:
- 1 can (5 oz) tuna, drained
- 1/4 cup diced celery
- 1/4 cup diced red onion
- 2 tablespoons plain Greek yogurt
- 1 tablespoon lemon juice
- Salt and pepper to taste
- Lettuce leaves for wrapping

Instructions:
1. In a bowl, combine tuna, celery, red onion, Greek yogurt, lemon juice, salt, and pepper.
2. Spoon the tuna salad into lettuce leaves and wrap.

Nutritional Info: (per serving)
- Calories: 200
- Protein: 20g
- Fat: 5g
- Carbohydrates: 10g
- Fiber: 3g

Prep Time: 10 minutes
Cook Time: 0 minutes
Serving: 2

---

13. VEGETABLE AND BEAN SOUP

Ingredients:
- 1 tablespoon olive oil
- 1/2 onion, chopped
- 2 garlic cloves, minced
- 1 carrot, diced
- 1 celery stalk, diced
- 1 can (15 oz) diced tomatoes
- 4 cups vegetable broth
- 1 can (15 oz) white beans, drained and rinsed
- 1 teaspoon dried thyme
- Salt and pepper to taste
- Fresh parsley for garnish

Instructions:
1. Heat olive oil in a large pot over medium heat. Add onion and garlic, and sauté until softened.
2. Add carrot and celery, and cook for another 5 minutes.
3. Stir in diced tomatoes, vegetable broth, white beans, thyme, salt, and pepper. Bring to a simmer.
4. Cook for 20-30 minutes, or until vegetables are tender.
5. Garnish with fresh parsley before serving.

Nutritional Info: (per serving)
- Calories: 250
- Protein: 10g
- Fat: 5g
- Carbohydrates: 40g
- Fiber: 10g

Prep Time: 10 minutes
Cook Time: 30 minutes
Serving: 4

---

14. CHICKEN AND AVOCADO SALAD

Ingredients:
- 1 cooked chicken breast, shredded
- 1 avocado, diced
- 1/4 cup diced red onion
- 1/4 cup diced bell pepper
- 1/4 cup diced cucumber
- 2 tablespoons plain Greek yogurt
- 1 tablespoon lemon juice
- Salt and pepper to taste
- Mixed greens for serving

Instructions:
1. In a bowl, combine shredded chicken breast, diced avocado, red onion, bell pepper, and cucumber.
2. In a small bowl, mix together Greek yogurt, lemon juice, salt, and pepper. Pour over the chicken mixture and toss to coat.
3. Serve over mixed greens.

Nutritional Info: (per serving)
- Calories: 300
- Protein: 25g
- Fat: 15g
- Carbohydrates: 15g
- Fiber: 7g

Prep Time: 10 minutes
Cook Time: 0 minutes
Serving: 1

---

15. EGGPLANT AND CHICKPEA CURRY

Ingredients:
- 1 tablespoon olive oil
- 1/2 onion, chopped
- 2 garlic cloves, minced
- 1 eggplant, diced
- 1 can (15 oz) chickpeas, drained and rinsed
- 1 can (15 oz) diced tomatoes
- 1 can (15 oz) coconut milk
- 2 tablespoons curry powder
- Salt and pepper to taste
- Cooked brown rice for serving

Instructions:
1. Heat olive oil in a large skillet over medium heat. Add onion and garlic, and sauté until softened.
2. Add diced eggplant and cook for 5-7 minutes, or until softened.
3. Stir in chickpeas, diced tomatoes, coconut milk, curry powder, salt, and pepper. Bring to a simmer.
4. Cook for 15-20 minutes, stirring occasionally.
5. Serve over cooked brown rice.

Nutritional Info: (per serving)
- Calories: 400
- Protein: 15g
- Fat: 20g
- Carbohydrates: 45g
- Fiber: 10g

Prep Time: 15 minutes
Cook Time: 25 minutes
Serving: 4

---

16. CHICKEN AND VEGETABLE STIR-FRY

Ingredients:
- 1 tablespoon olive oil
- 1/2 onion, chopped
- 2 garlic cloves, minced
- 1/2 cup sliced carrots
- 1/2 cup broccoli florets
- 1/2 cup sliced bell peppers
- 1/2 cup sliced mushrooms
- 1/2 cup snap peas
- 1 small chicken breast, cooked and sliced
- 2 tablespoons soy sauce

- 1 tablespoon honey
- Cooked brown rice for serving

Instructions:
1. Heat olive oil in a large skillet over medium heat. Add onion and garlic, and sauté for 1 minute.
2. Add carrots, broccoli, bell peppers, mushrooms, and snap peas. Cook, stirring occasionally, until vegetables are tender-crisp.
3. Add sliced chicken breast, soy sauce, and honey. Cook for another 2-3 minutes, stirring gently.
4. Serve over cooked brown rice.

Nutritional Info: (per serving)
- Calories: 400
- Protein: 25g
- Fat: 15g
- Carbohydrates: 40g
- Fiber: 6g

Prep Time: 15 minutes
Cook Time: 15 minutes
Serving: 1

---

17. TUNA SALAD LETTUCE WRAPS

Ingredients:
- 1 can (5 oz) tuna, drained
- 1/4 cup diced celery
- 1/4 cup diced red onion
- 2 tablespoons plain Greek yogurt
- 1 tablespoon lemon juice
- Salt and pepper to taste
- Lettuce leaves for wrapping

Instructions:
1. In a bowl, combine tuna, celery, red onion, Greek yogurt, lemon juice, salt, and pepper.
2. Spoon the tuna salad into lettuce leaves and wrap.

Nutritional Info: (per serving)
- Calories: 200
- Protein: 20g
- Fat: 5g
- Carbohydrates: 10g
- Fiber: 3g

Prep Time: 10 minutes
Cook Time: 0 minutes
Serving: 2

---

18. CHICKEN AND VEGETABLE SOUP

Ingredients:
- 1 tablespoon olive oil
- 1/2 onion, chopped
- 2 garlic cloves, minced
- 1 carrot, diced
- 1 celery stalk, diced
- 4 cups chicken broth
- 1 cup diced cooked chicken breast
- 1/2 cup frozen peas
- Salt and pepper to taste
- Fresh parsley for garnish

Instructions:
1. Heat olive oil in a large pot over medium heat. Add onion and garlic, and sauté until softened.
2. Add carrot and celery, and cook for another 5 minutes.
3. Pour in chicken broth and bring to a simmer.
4. Add chicken breast and frozen peas. Cook for another 5 minutes, or until heated through.
5. Season with salt and pepper. Garnish with fresh parsley before serving.

Nutritional Info: (per serving)
- Calories: 250
- Protein: 20g
- Fat: 10g
- Carbohydrates: 20g
- Fiber: 4g

Prep Time: 10 minutes
Cook Time: 20 minutes
Serving: 4

---

19. MEDITERRANEAN CHICKPEA SALAD

Ingredients:
- 1 can (15 oz) chickpeas, drained and rinsed
- 1/2 cucumber, diced
- 1/2 cup cherry tomatoes, halved
- 1/4 cup diced red onion
- 1/4 cup chopped fresh parsley
- Juice of 1 lemon
- 2 tablespoons olive oil
- Salt and pepper to taste
- Crumbled feta cheese (optional)

Instructions:
1. In a large bowl, combine chickpeas, cucumber, cherry tomatoes, red onion, and parsley.
2. In a small bowl, whisk together lemon juice, olive oil, salt, and pepper.
3. Pour the dressing over the salad and toss to coat.
4. Sprinkle with crumbled feta cheese if desired.

Nutritional Info: (per serving)
- Calories: 350
- Protein: 10g
- Fat: 20g
- Carbohydrates: 30g
- Fiber: 5g

Prep Time: 10 minutes
Cook Time: 0 minutes
Serving: 2

---

20. SWEET POTATO AND BLACK BEAN QUESADILLAS

Ingredients:
- 1 large sweet potato, peeled and diced
- 1 can (15 oz) black beans, drained and rinsed
- 1 teaspoon cumin
- 1/2 teaspoon chili powder
- Salt and pepper to taste
- 4 whole wheat tortillas
- 1 cup shredded cheese (such as cheddar or Monterey Jack)
- Salsa and Greek yogurt for serving

Instructions:
1. Steam or microwave the sweet potato until tender. Mash with a fork.

2. In a bowl, combine mashed sweet potato, black beans, cumin, chili powder, salt, and pepper.
3. Divide the mixture evenly among 2 tortillas. Top each with 1/2 cup shredded cheese and another tortilla.
4. Heat a large skillet over medium heat. Cook each quesadilla for 3-4 minutes per side, or until the cheese is melted and the tortillas are crispy.
5. Cut into wedges and serve with salsa and Greek yogurt.

Nutritional Info: (per serving)
- Calories: 400
- Protein: 20g
- Fat: 15g
- Carbohydrates: 50g
- Fiber: 10g

Prep Time: 15 minutes
Cook Time: 15 minutes
Serving: 2

Chapter 4: Dinner Recipes

1. SPINACH AND MUSHROOM STUFFED CHICKEN

Ingredients:
- 4 chicken breasts
- 2 cups chopped spinach
- 1 cup sliced mushrooms
- 1/2 cup shredded mozzarella cheese
- 1/4 cup grated Parmesan cheese
- 2 garlic cloves, minced
- 1 teaspoon olive oil
- Salt and pepper to taste

Instructions:
1. Preheat the oven to 375°F (190°C).
2. In a skillet, heat olive oil over medium heat. Add garlic, spinach, and mushrooms. Cook until spinach is wilted and mushrooms are tender. Remove from heat and let cool.
3. Butterfly each chicken breast and stuff with the spinach-mushroom mixture.
4. Place stuffed chicken breasts in a baking dish. Season with salt and pepper.
5. Sprinkle mozzarella and Parmesan cheese over the chicken.
6. Bake for 25-30 minutes, or until chicken is cooked through.

Nutritional Info: (per serving)
- Calories: 300
- Protein: 40g
- Fat: 12g
- Carbohydrates: 4g
- Fiber: 2g

Prep Time: 15 minutes
Cook Time: 30 minutes

Serving: 4

---

2. SALMON AND VEGETABLE SHEET PAN DINNER

Ingredients:
- 4 salmon filets
- 2 cups broccoli florets
- 1 red bell pepper, sliced
- 1 yellow bell pepper, sliced
- 1/2 red onion, sliced
- 2 tablespoons olive oil
- 2 tablespoons lemon juice
- 2 teaspoons Italian seasoning
- Salt and pepper to taste

Instructions:
1. Preheat the oven to 400°F (200°C).
2. Place salmon filets on one side of a large baking sheet.
3. On the other side of the baking sheet, arrange broccoli, bell peppers, and onion slices.
4. Drizzle olive oil and lemon juice over everything. Sprinkle with Italian seasoning, salt, and pepper.
5. Bake for 15-20 minutes, or until salmon is cooked through and vegetables are tender.

Nutritional Info: (per serving)
- Calories: 350
- Protein: 30g
- Fat: 20g
- Carbohydrates: 12g
- Fiber: 4g

Prep Time: 10 minutes

Cook Time: 20 minutes
Serving: 4

---

3. TURKEY AND QUINOA STUFFED PEPPERS

Ingredients:
- 4 bell peppers, halved and seeded
- 1 pound ground turkey
- 1 cup cooked quinoa
- 1 can (15 oz) black beans, drained and rinsed
- 1 can (15 oz) diced tomatoes
- 1 tablespoon chili powder
- 1 teaspoon cumin
- Salt and pepper to taste
- 1/2 cup shredded cheddar cheese

Instructions:
1. Preheat the oven to 375°F (190°C).
2. In a skillet, cook ground turkey until browned. Drain any excess fat.
3. Stir in cooked quinoa, black beans, diced tomatoes, chili powder, cumin, salt, and pepper.
4. Spoon the turkey-quinoa mixture into each bell pepper half.
5. Place stuffed peppers in a baking dish. Cover with foil and bake for 30 minutes.
6. Remove foil, sprinkle cheddar cheese over the peppers, and bake for an additional 10 minutes, or until the cheese is melted and bubbly.

Nutritional Info: (per serving)
- Calories: 350
- Protein: 30g
- Fat: 10g
- Carbohydrates: 35g
- Fiber: 10g

Prep Time: 20 minutes
Cook Time: 40 minutes
Serving: 4

---

4. CHICKEN AND BROCCOLI CASSEROLE

Ingredients:
- 2 cups cooked shredded chicken
- 4 cups broccoli florets, steamed
- 1 cup plain Greek yogurt
- 1/2 cup grated Parmesan cheese
- 1/2 cup shredded mozzarella cheese
- 2 garlic cloves, minced
- 1 teaspoon Italian seasoning
- Salt and pepper to taste
- 1/2 cup breadcrumbs (optional)

Instructions:
1. Preheat the oven to 375°F (190°C). Grease a baking dish.
2. In a large bowl, combine chicken, steamed broccoli, Greek yogurt, Parmesan cheese, mozzarella cheese, garlic, Italian seasoning, salt, and pepper.
3. Spread the mixture evenly in the prepared baking dish.
4. Sprinkle bread crumbs over the top (if using).
5. Bake for 25-30 minutes, or until bubbly and golden brown.

Nutritional Info: (per serving)
- Calories: 300
- Protein: 40g
- Fat: 10g
- Carbohydrates: 15g
- Fiber: 5g

Prep Time: 15 minutes
Cook Time: 30 minutes
Serving: 4

---

5. VEGETABLE AND CHICKPEA CURRY

Ingredients:
- 1 tablespoon olive oil
- 1/2 onion, chopped
- 2 garlic cloves, minced
- 1 tablespoon grated ginger
- 1 tablespoon curry powder
- 1 can (15 oz) chickpeas, drained and rinsed
- 1 can (15 oz) diced tomatoes
- 1 can (15 oz) coconut milk
- 2 cups chopped vegetables (such as bell peppers, zucchini, and carrots)
- Salt and pepper to taste
- Cooked brown rice for serving

Instructions:
1. Heat olive oil in a large skillet over medium heat. Add onion, garlic, and ginger. Sauté for 2-3 minutes.
2. Stir in curry powder and cook for another minute.
3. Add chickpeas, diced tomatoes, coconut milk, and vegetables. Bring to a simmer.
4. Cook for 15-20 minutes, or until vegetables are tender.
5. Season with salt and pepper. Serve over cooked brown rice.

Nutritional Info: (per serving)
- Calories: 400
- Protein: 15g
- Fat: 20g

- Carbohydrates: 45g
- Fiber: 10g

Prep Time: 15 minutes
Cook Time: 25 minutes
Serving: 4

---

6. BAKED SALMON WITH ASPARAGUS

Ingredients:
- 4 salmon filets
- 1 bunch asparagus, trimmed
- 2 tablespoons olive oil
- 2 tablespoons lemon juice
- 2 garlic cloves, minced
- 1 teaspoon dried dill
- Salt and pepper to taste

Instructions:
1. Preheat the oven to 400°F (200°C). Grease a baking dish.
2. Place salmon filets in the prepared baking dish. Arrange asparagus around the salmon.
3. In a small bowl, whisk together olive oil, lemon juice, garlic, dill, salt, and pepper.
4. Pour the mixture over the salmon and asparagus.
5. Bake for 12-15 minutes, or until salmon is cooked through and flakes easily with a fork.

Nutritional Info: (per serving)
- Calories: 350
- Protein: 30g
- Fat: 20g
- Carbohydrates: 10g

- Fiber: 4g

Prep Time: 10 minutes
Cook Time: 15 minutes
Serving: 4

---

7. QUINOA AND BLACK BEAN STUFFED SWEET POTATOES

Ingredients:
- 4 medium sweet potatoes
- 1 can (15 oz) black beans, drained and rinsed
- 1 cup cooked quinoa
- 1/2 cup diced bell peppers
- 1/2 cup diced red onion
- 1/2 cup corn kernels
- 1 teaspoon cumin
- 1/2 teaspoon chili powder
- Salt and pepper to taste
- Fresh cilantro for garnish

Instructions:
1. Preheat the oven to 400°F (200°C).
2. Pierce sweet potatoes with a fork and place them on a baking sheet. Bake for 45-60 minutes, or until tender.
3. In a large bowl, combine black beans, quinoa, bell peppers, red onion, corn, cumin, chili powder, salt, and pepper.
4. Cut a slit in each sweet potato and fluff the flesh with a fork.
5. Spoon the black bean-quinoa mixture into each sweet potato.
6. Garnish with fresh cilantro before serving.

Nutritional Info: (per serving)
- Calories: 350
- Protein: 15g

- Fat: 5g
- Carbohydrates: 70g
- Fiber: 12g

Prep Time: 10 minutes
Cook Time: 60 minutes
Serving: 4

---

8. TURKEY AND VEGETABLE SKILLET

Ingredients:
- 1 pound ground turkey
- 1 onion, chopped
- 2 garlic cloves, minced
- 1 zucchini, diced
- 1 bell pepper, diced
- 1 can (15 oz) diced tomatoes
- 1 teaspoon Italian seasoning
- Salt and pepper to taste
- Fresh basil for garnish

Instructions:
1. In a large skillet, cook ground turkey over medium heat until browned.
2. Add onion and garlic, and cook for another 2-3 minutes.
3. Stir in zucchini, bell pepper, diced tomatoes, Italian seasoning, salt, and pepper.
4. Simmer for 10-15 minutes, or until vegetables are tender and flavors are blended.
5. Garnish with fresh basil before serving.

Nutritional Info: (per serving)
- Calories: 300
- Protein: 25g

- Fat: 10g
- Carbohydrates: 20g
- Fiber: 5g

Prep Time: 10 minutes
Cook Time: 20 minutes
Serving: 4

---

9. EGGPLANT AND ZUCCHINI LASAGNA

Ingredients:
- 1 large eggplant, sliced lengthwise
- 2 zucchinis, sliced lengthwise
- 2 cups marinara sauce
- 1 cup ricotta cheese
- 1 cup shredded mozzarella cheese
- 1/4 cup grated Parmesan cheese
- 1 teaspoon dried oregano
- Salt and pepper to taste
- Fresh basil for garnish

Instructions:
1. Preheat the oven to 375°F (190°C). Grease a baking dish.
2. Place a layer of eggplant slices on the bottom of the baking dish.
3. Spread half of the marinara sauce over the eggplant slices.
4. Arrange a layer of zucchini slices over the marinara sauce.
5. In a bowl, combine ricotta cheese, mozzarella cheese, Parmesan cheese, oregano, salt, and pepper.
6. Spread half of the cheese mixture over the zucchini slices.
7. Repeat the layers: eggplant, marinara sauce, zucchini, cheese mixture.
8. Cover the baking dish with foil and bake for 30 minutes.
9. Remove foil and bake for an additional 15 minutes, or until bubbly and golden.

10. Garnish with fresh basil before serving.

Nutritional Info: (per serving)
- Calories: 350
- Protein: 20g
- Fat: 15g
- Carbohydrates: 30g
- Fiber: 10g

Prep Time: 20 minutes
Cook Time: 45 minutes
Serving: 4

---

10. MEXICAN QUINOA CASSEROLE

Ingredients:
- 1 cup uncooked quinoa
- 1 can (15 oz) black beans, drained and rinsed
- 1 can (15 oz) diced tomatoes
- 1 cup frozen corn kernels
- 1 bell pepper, diced
- 1 onion, chopped
- 2 garlic cloves, minced
- 1 teaspoon cumin
- 1 teaspoon chili powder
- 1/2 teaspoon paprika
- Salt and pepper to taste
- 1 cup shredded cheddar cheese
- Fresh cilantro for garnish

Instructions:
1. Preheat the oven to 375°F (190°C). Grease a baking dish.
2. Cook quinoa according to package instructions.

3. In a large bowl, combine cooked quinoa, black beans, diced tomatoes, corn, bell pepper, onion, garlic, cumin, chili powder, paprika, salt, and pepper.
4. Spread the mixture evenly in the prepared baking dish.
5. Top with shredded cheddar cheese.
6. Cover with foil and bake for 20 minutes.
7. Remove foil and bake for an additional 10 minutes, or until the cheese is melted and bubbly.
8. Garnish with fresh cilantro before serving.

Nutritional Info: (per serving)
- Calories: 400
- Protein: 20g
- Fat: 15g
- Carbohydrates: 50g
- Fiber: 10g

Prep Time: 15 minutes
Cook Time: 30 minutes
Serving: 4

---

11. SLOW COOKER CHICKEN AND VEGETABLE STEW

Ingredients:
- 1 pound boneless, skinless chicken thighs
- 4 cups chicken broth
- 2 carrots, sliced
- 2 celery stalks, sliced
- 1 onion, chopped
- 2 garlic cloves, minced
- 1 teaspoon dried thyme
- 1 teaspoon dried rosemary
- Salt and pepper to taste

- 2 cups baby spinach

Instructions:
1. Place chicken thighs in a slow cooker. Add chicken broth, carrots, celery, onion, garlic, thyme, rosemary, salt, and pepper.
2. Cover and cook on low for 6-8 hours or high for 3-4 hours, or until chicken is tender.
3. Remove chicken from the slow cooker and shred with two forks. Return chicken to the slow cooker.
4. Stir in baby spinach and cook for an additional 10 minutes, or until spinach is wilted.
5. Serve hot.

Nutritional Info: (per serving)
- Calories: 300
- Protein: 30g
- Fat: 10g
- Carbohydrates: 20g
- Fiber: 5g

Prep Time: 15 minutes
Cook Time: 6-8 hours (slow cooker)
Serving: 4

---

12. TURKEY AND VEGETABLE STIR-FRY

Ingredients:
- 1 pound ground turkey
- 1 tablespoon olive oil
- 1 onion, chopped
- 2 garlic cloves, minced
- 1 bell pepper, sliced
- 1 zucchini, sliced

- 1 cup snap peas
- 1/4 cup soy sauce
- 2 tablespoons hoisin sauce
- 1 tablespoon sesame oil
- Cooked brown rice for serving

Instructions:
1. In a large skillet, heat olive oil over medium heat. Add ground turkey and cook until browned.
2. Add onion and garlic, and cook for another 2-3 minutes.
3. Stir in bell pepper, zucchini, and snap peas. Cook for 5-7 minutes, or until vegetables are tender-crisp.
4. In a small bowl, whisk together soy sauce, hoisin sauce, and sesame oil. Pour over the turkey and vegetables. Cook for another 2-3 minutes, stirring gently.
5. Serve over cooked brown rice.

Nutritional Info: (per serving)
- Calories: 350
- Protein: 30g
- Fat: 15g
- Carbohydrates: 25g
- Fiber: 5g

Prep Time: 15 minutes
Cook Time: 20 minutes
Serving: 4

---

13. VEGETABLE AND CHICKEN QUINOA BAKE

Ingredients:
- 1 cup uncooked quinoa
- 2 cups chicken broth

- 1 pound boneless, skinless chicken breasts, diced
- 1 onion, chopped
- 2 garlic cloves, minced
- 1 red bell pepper, chopped
- 1 yellow bell pepper, chopped
- 1 zucchini, chopped
- 1 can (15 oz) diced tomatoes
- 1 teaspoon dried oregano
- 1 teaspoon dried basil
- Salt and pepper to taste
- 1/2 cup shredded mozzarella cheese

Instructions:
1. Preheat the oven to 375°F (190°C). Grease a baking dish.
2. In a large skillet, combine quinoa and chicken broth. Bring to a boil, then reduce heat and simmer for 10 minutes.
3. Add diced chicken, onion, garlic, bell peppers, zucchini, diced tomatoes, oregano, basil, salt, and pepper to the skillet. Stir to combine.
4. Transfer the mixture to the prepared baking dish. Cover with foil and bake for 30 minutes.
5. Remove foil, sprinkle mozzarella cheese over the top, and bake for an additional 10 minutes, or until the cheese is melted and bubbly.
6. Serve hot.

Nutritional Info: (per serving)
- Calories: 400
- Protein: 30g
- Fat: 10g
- Carbohydrates: 45g
- Fiber: 7g

Prep Time: 15 minutes
Cook Time: 40 minutes
Serving: 4

---

14. BEEF AND BROCCOLI STIR-FRY

Ingredients:
- 1 pound flank steak, thinly sliced
- 1/4 cup soy sauce
- 2 tablespoons oyster sauce
- 1 tablespoon sesame oil
- 2 garlic cloves, minced
- 1 teaspoon grated ginger
- 2 cups broccoli florets
- 1 red bell pepper, sliced
- 1/2 onion, sliced
- Cooked brown rice for serving

Instructions:
1. In a bowl, combine soy sauce, oyster sauce, sesame oil, garlic, and ginger. Add sliced flank steak and marinate for 15-30 minutes.
2. Heat a large skillet over medium-high heat. AddI'm glad to continue! Here are more dinner recipes for your Alzheimer's cookbook:

---

15. SWEET POTATO AND CHICKPEA CURRY

Ingredients:
- 2 tablespoons olive oil
- 1 onion, chopped
- 2 garlic cloves, minced
- 1 tablespoon grated ginger
- 2 tablespoons curry powder
- 1 teaspoon ground cumin
- 1 teaspoon ground coriander
- 1/2 teaspoon turmeric

- 1 can (15 oz) chickpeas, drained and rinsed
- 1 large sweet potato, peeled and diced
- 1 can (14 oz) coconut milk
- 1 cup vegetable broth
- Salt and pepper to taste
- Fresh cilantro for garnish

Instructions:
1. In a large pot, heat olive oil over medium heat. Add onion, garlic, and ginger. Sauté for 2-3 minutes.
2. Stir in curry powder, cumin, coriander, and turmeric. Cook for another minute.
3. Add chickpeas, sweet potato, coconut milk, and vegetable broth. Bring to a simmer.
4. Cook for 20-25 minutes, or until sweet potatoes are tender.
5. Season with salt and pepper. Garnish with fresh cilantro before serving.

Nutritional Info: (per serving)
- Calories: 400
- Protein: 10g
- Fat: 20g
- Carbohydrates: 45g
- Fiber: 10g

Prep Time: 15 minutes
Cook Time: 25 minutes
Serving: 4

---

16. TURKEY MEATBALLS WITH ZUCCHINI NOODLES

Ingredients:
- 1 pound ground turkey
- 1/2 cup breadcrumbs

- 1/4 cup grated Parmesan cheese
- 1 egg
- 2 garlic cloves, minced
- 1 teaspoon dried oregano
- Salt and pepper to taste
- 2 zucchinis, spiralized into noodles
- 1 can (14 oz) diced tomatoes
- 1 teaspoon Italian seasoning
- Fresh basil for garnish

Instructions:
1. Preheat the oven to 400°F (200°C). Line a baking sheet with parchment paper.
2. In a large bowl, combine ground turkey, breadcrumbs, Parmesan cheese, egg, garlic, oregano, salt, and pepper. Mix until well combined.
3. Shape the mixture into meatballs and place them on the prepared baking sheet.
4. Bake for 15-20 minutes, or until cooked through.
5. In a large skillet, heat diced tomatoes and Italian seasoning over medium heat. Add zucchini noodles and cook for 5-7 minutes, or until noodles are tender.
6. Serve turkey meatballs over zucchini noodles. Garnish with fresh basil.

Nutritional Info: (per serving)
- Calories: 350
- Protein: 30g
- Fat: 15g
- Carbohydrates: 20g
- Fiber: 5g

Prep Time: 15 minutes
Cook Time: 25 minutes
Serving: 4

---

17. LEMON GARLIC SHRIMP WITH BROCCOLI

Ingredients:
- 1 pound shrimp, peeled and deveined
- 2 tablespoons olive oil
- 2 garlic cloves, minced
- Zest of 1 lemon
- Juice of 1 lemon
- 1 teaspoon dried thyme
- Salt and pepper to taste
- 4 cups broccoli florets

Instructions:
1. In a large bowl, combine shrimp, olive oil, garlic, lemon zest, lemon juice, thyme, salt, and pepper. Mix until shrimp are coated.
2. Heat a large skillet over medium-high heat. Add shrimp and cook for 2-3 minutes per side, or until pink and cooked through. Remove shrimp from skillet and set aside.
3. In the same skillet, add broccoli florets and cook for 5-7 minutes, or until tender-crisp.
4. Serve shrimp over broccoli.

Nutritional Info: (per serving)
- Calories: 300
- Protein: 30g
- Fat: 15g
- Carbohydrates: 15g
- Fiber: 5g

Prep Time: 10 minutes
Cook Time: 15 minutes
Serving: 4

---

18. CHICKEN AND VEGETABLE STIR-FRY

Ingredients:
- 1 pound boneless, skinless chicken breasts, cut into strips
- 2 tablespoons soy sauce
- 1 tablespoon hoisin sauce
- 1 tablespoon oyster sauce
- 1 teaspoon sesame oil
- 2 tablespoons olive oil
- 2 garlic cloves, minced
- 1 bell pepper, sliced
- 1 cup snap peas
- 1 cup broccoli florets
- 1/2 onion, sliced
- Cooked brown rice for serving

Instructions:
1. In a bowl, combine chicken strips, soy sauce, hoisin sauce, oyster sauce, and sesame oil. Mix until chicken is coated. Marinate for 15-20 minutes.
2. Heat olive oil in a large skillet over medium-high heat. Add garlic and cook for 1 minute.
3. Add marinated chicken strips to the skillet. Cook for 5-7 minutes, or until chicken is cooked through.
4. Add bell pepper, snap peas, broccoli florets, and onion to the skillet. Cook for another 5 minutes, or until vegetables are tender-crisp.
5. Serve stir-fry over cooked brown rice.

Nutritional Info: (per serving)
- Calories: 350
- Protein: 30g
- Fat: 15g
- Carbohydrates: 25g
- Fiber: 5g

Prep Time: 15 minutes

Cook Time: 15 minutes
Serving: 4

---

19. BAKED CHICKEN PARMESAN

Ingredients:
- 4 boneless, skinless chicken breasts
- 1 cup breadcrumbs
- 1/2 cup grated Parmesan cheese
- 1 teaspoon Italian seasoning
- Salt and pepper to taste
- 1 egg, beaten
- 1 cup marinara sauce
- 1 cup shredded mozzarella cheese
- Fresh basil for garnish

Instructions:
1. Preheat the oven to 400°F (200°C). Grease a baking dish.
2. In a shallow dish, combine breadcrumbs, Parmesan cheese, Italian seasoning, salt, and pepper.
3. Dip each chicken breast in beaten egg, then coat with breadcrumb mixture. Place chicken breasts in the prepared baking dish.
4. Bake for 20-25 minutes, or until chicken is cooked through.
5. Remove chicken from the oven and top each breast with marinara sauce and mozzarella cheese.
6. Return to the oven and bake for an additional 5-10 minutes, or until the cheese is melted and bubbly.
7. Garnish with fresh basil before serving.

Nutritional Info: (per serving)
- Calories: 350
- Protein: 40g
- Fat: 10g

- Carbohydrates: 20g
- Fiber: 2g

Prep Time: 15 minutes
Cook Time: 30 minutes
Serving: 4

---

20. ROASTED VEGETABLE AND CHICKPEA SALAD

Ingredients:
- 1 can (15 oz) chickpeas, drained and rinsed
- 2 cups mixed vegetables (such as bell peppers, zucchini, and cherry tomatoes), chopped
- 2 tablespoons olive oil
- 1 teaspoon cumin
- 1 teaspoon paprika
- Salt and pepper to taste
- 4 cups mixed greens
- 1/4 cup feta cheese, crumbled
- Balsamic glaze for drizzling

Instructions:
1. Preheat the oven to 400°F (200°C). Line a baking sheet with parchment paper.
2. In a bowl, combine chickpeas, mixed vegetables, olive oil, cumin, paprika, salt, and pepper. Mix until vegetables are coated.
3. Spread the mixture evenly on the prepared baking sheet.
4. Roast in the preheated oven for 25-30 minutes, or until vegetables are tender and chickpeas are crispy.
5. Divide mixed greens among serving plates. Top with roasted vegetable and chickpea mixture.
6. Sprinkle with crumbled feta cheese and drizzle with balsamic glaze before serving.

Nutritional Info: (per serving)
- Calories: 300
- Protein: 10g
- Fat: 15g
- Carbohydrates: 35g
- Fiber: 8g

Prep Time: 15 minutes
Cook Time: 30 minutes
Serving: 4

Chapter 5: Snacks and Desserts

1. ALMOND BUTTER ENERGY BALLS
   - Ingredients:
     - 1 cup almond butter
     - 1/2 cup honey
     - 1 teaspoon vanilla extract
     - 2 cups rolled oats
     - 1/2 cup mini chocolate chips
   - Instructions:
     1. In a bowl, mix almond butter, honey, and vanilla extract.
     2. Stir in oats and chocolate chips.
     3. Roll into balls and refrigerate for 30 minutes.

2. GREEK YOGURT BARK
   - Ingredients:
     - 2 cups Greek yogurt
     - 1/4 cup honey
     - 1/2 cup mixed berries
     - 1/4 cup granola
   - Instructions:
     1. Mix Greek yogurt and honey.
     2. Spread onto a baking sheet lined with parchment paper.
     3. Sprinkle it with berries and granola.
     4. Freeze for 2 hours, then break into pieces.

3. CARROT CAKE ENERGY BITES
   - Ingredients:
     - 1 cup shredded carrots
     - 1 cup oats
     - 1/2 cup dates, pitted
     - 1/2 cup almonds
     - 1 teaspoon cinnamon
     - 1/2 teaspoon nutmeg
   - Instructions:

1. Blend all ingredients in a food processor.
2. Roll into balls and refrigerate for 30 minutes.

4. SPINACH AND ARTICHOKE DIP
   - Ingredients:
     - 1 cup Greek yogurt
     - 1 cup chopped spinach
     - 1/2 cup chopped artichoke hearts
     - 1/4 cup grated Parmesan cheese
     - 1/4 teaspoon garlic powder
     - Salt and pepper to taste
   - Instructions:
     1. Mix all ingredients in a bowl.
     2. Serve with whole grain crackers or vegetable sticks.

5. TURMERIC ROASTED CHICKPEAS
   - Ingredients:
     - 1 can (15 oz) chickpeas, drained and rinsed
     - 1 tablespoon olive oil
     - 1 teaspoon turmeric
     - 1/2 teaspoon cumin
     - Salt to taste
   - Instructions:
     1. Preheat the oven to 400°F (200°C).
     2. Toss chickpeas with olive oil, turmeric, cumin, and salt.
     3. Spread on a baking sheet and roast for 20-25 minutes, shaking halfway through.

6. COCONUT CHIA PUDDING
   - Ingredients:
     - 1/4 cup chia seeds
     - 1 cup coconut milk
     - 1 tablespoon honey
     - 1/2 teaspoon vanilla extract
   - Instructions:

1. Mix chia seeds, coconut milk, honey, and vanilla extract in a bowl.
   2. Refrigerate for at least 2 hours, or until thickened.
   3. Serve with fresh berries.

7. APPLE SANDWICHES
   - Ingredients:
     - 1 apple, cored and sliced
     - 2 tablespoons almond butter
     - Granola for topping
   - Instructions:
     1. Spread almond butter on apple slices.
     2. Sprinkle granola and sandwich together.

8. CHIA SEED PUDDING
   - Ingredients:
     - 2 tablespoons chia seeds
     - 1/2 cup almond milk
     - 1/2 teaspoon vanilla extract
     - 1 tablespoon honey
   - Instructions:
     1. Mix chia seeds, almond milk, vanilla extract, and honey in a bowl.
     2. Refrigerate for at least 2 hours, or until thickened.
     3. Serve with sliced fruit.

9. QUINOA FRUIT SALAD
   - Ingredients:
     - 1/2 cup cooked quinoa
     - 1/2 cup mixed berries
     - 1/4 cup chopped nuts
     - 1 tablespoon honey
   - Instructions:
     1. Mix quinoa, mixed berries, chopped nuts, and honey in a bowl.
     2. Serve chilled.

10. STUFFED DATES
    - Ingredients:
        - 10 dates, pitted
        - 2 tablespoons almond butter
        - 10 almonds
    - Instructions:
        1. Fill each date with almond butter.
        2. Press an almond into the almond butter.

11. VEGGIE WRAP
    - Ingredients:
        - 1 whole grain wrap
        - 2 tablespoons hummus
        - Sliced cucumber, bell pepper, and carrot
    - Instructions:
        1. Spread hummus on the wrap.
        2. Layer with sliced vegetables and roll up.

12. COTTAGE CHEESE WITH FRUIT
    - Ingredients:
        - 1/2 cup cottage cheese
        - 1/2 cup mixed berries
        - 1 tablespoon honey
    - Instructions:
        1. Mix cottage cheese, mixed berries, and honey in a bowl.
        2. Serve chilled.

13. AVOCADO TOAST
    - Ingredients:
        - 1 slice whole grain bread, toasted
        - 1/2 avocado, mashed
        - Sliced tomato
        - Sprouts
        - Salt and pepper to taste
    - Instructions:

1. Spread mashed avocado on toasted bread.
2. Top with sliced tomato and sprouts.
3. Season with salt and pepper.

14. RICE CAKES WITH HUMMUS AND CUCUMBER
    - Ingredients:
        - 2 rice cakes
        - 2 tablespoons hummus
        - Sliced cucumber
    - Instructions:
        1. Spread hummus on rice cakes.
        2. Top with sliced cucumber.

15. CUCUMBER BITES
    - Ingredients:
        - 1 cucumber, sliced
        - 1/2 cup Greek yogurt
        - 1/4 cup chopped fresh dill
        - Salt and pepper to taste
    - Instructions:
        1. Mix Greek yogurt, chopped dill, salt, and pepper in a bowl.
        2. Top cucumber slices with yogurt mixture.

16. BERRY SMOOTHIE
    - Ingredients:
        - 1/2 cup mixed berries
        - 1/2 banana
        - 1/2 cup Greek yogurt
        - 1/2 cup almond milk
        - 1 tablespoon honey
    - Instructions:
        1. Blend mixed berries, banana, Greek yogurt, almond milk, and honey until smooth.

17. STUFFED MINI PEPPERS
- Ingredients:
  - 10 mini bell peppers, halved and seeded
  - 1/2 cup cream cheese
  - 1/4 cup chopped chives
  - Salt and pepper to taste
- Instructions:
  1. Mix cream cheese, chopped chives, salt, and pepper in a bowl.
  2. Fill each mini pepper half with the cream cheese mixture.

18. GREEK YOGURT DIP WITH VEGGIE STICKS
- Ingredients:
  - 1 cup Greek yogurt
  - 1 tablespoon lemon juice
  - 1 teaspoon dried dill
  - Salt and pepper to taste
  - Assorted vegetable sticks (carrots, celery, bell peppers)
- Instructions:
  1. Mix Greek yogurt, lemon juice, dried dill, salt, and pepper in a bowl.
  2. Serve with vegetable sticks.

19. CHOCOLATE AVOCADO MOUSSE
- Ingredients:
  - 2 ripe avocados
  - 1/4 cup cocoa powder
  - 1/4 cup honey
  - 1/2 teaspoon vanilla extract
- Instructions:
  1. Blend avocados, cocoa powder, honey, and vanilla extract until smooth.
  2. Serve chilled.

20. APPLE NACHOS
- Ingredients:
  - 1 apple, thinly sliced

- 2 tablespoons almond butter
- 2 tablespoons granola
- 1 tablespoon mini chocolate chips

- Instructions:
  1. Arrange apple slices on a plate.
  2. Drizzle almond butter over the apple slices.
  3. Sprinkle it with granola and mini chocolate chips.

Chapter 6: Caregiver Support

Tips for Caregivers

1. Establish a Routine: Maintain a consistent daily schedule for meals, medication, and activities to provide a sense of stability for the person with Alzheimer's.

2. Encourage Independence: Allow the person with Alzheimer's to do tasks on their own as much as possible, but be ready to offer assistance when needed.

3. Create a Safe Environment: Remove hazards such as loose rugs or clutter, install grab bars in the bathroom, and ensure that the home is well-lit to prevent falls.

4. Communicate Effectively: Use simple sentences and clear, concise instructions. Speak slowly and calmly, and allow time for the person to respond.

5. Provide Nutritious Meals: Offer a balanced diet rich in fruits, vegetables, whole grains, and lean proteins to support overall health and brain function.

6. Stay Active: Engage in physical activities together, such as walking or gentle stretching, to promote physical health and well-being.

7. Manage Medications: Keep track of medications and ensure they are taken as prescribed. Use pill organizers or reminders if needed.

8. Seek Support: Join a caregiver support group or seek counseling to manage stress and connect with others facing similar challenges.

9. Practice Self-Care: Take breaks when needed, prioritize your own health, and seek help from friends, family, or professional caregivers when necessary.

10. Be Patient and Flexible: Alzheimer's can be unpredictable, so approach each day with patience and a willingness to adapt to the person's changing needs.

These tips can help caregivers provide the best possible care for their loved ones with Alzheimer's while also taking care of themselves.

Self-Care for Caregivers

Self-care is crucial for caregivers to maintain their own physical and mental well-being while caring for someone with Alzheimer's. Here are some self-care tips for caregivers:

1. Take Breaks: It's important to take regular breaks to rest and recharge. Arrange for respite care or ask family and friends to help so you can have some time for yourself.

2. Prioritize Sleep: Getting enough rest is essential for your health. Try to maintain a regular sleep schedule and create a relaxing bedtime routine.

3. Eat Well: Proper nutrition is key to maintaining your energy levels and overall health. Eat a balanced diet rich in fruits, vegetables, whole grains, and lean proteins.

4. Stay Active: Regular physical activity can help reduce stress and improve your mood. Find activities you enjoy, such as walking, yoga, or swimming.

5. Connect with Others: Stay connected with friends, family, and support groups. Talking to others who understand what you're going through can provide comfort and encouragement.

6. Seek Help: Don't hesitate to ask for help when you need it. Whether it's assistance with caregiving duties or emotional support, reach out to others for help.

7. Manage Stress: Practice stress-relieving techniques such as deep breathing, meditation, or mindfulness to help manage stress and anxiety.

8. Set Realistic Expectations: Understand that you can't do everything perfectly. Set realistic expectations for yourself and prioritize tasks based on importance.

9. Maintain Hobbies and Interests: Make time for activities you enjoy, whether it's reading, gardening, or crafting. Engaging in hobbies can provide a much-needed break from caregiving duties.

10. Attend to Your Emotional Needs: Acknowledge and validate your feelings. It's normal to experience a range of emotions, including guilt, frustration, and sadness. Consider talking to a therapist or counselor for additional support.

By prioritizing self-care, caregivers can better manage the demands of caregiving and maintain their own health and well-being.

Chapter 7: 28-Day Meal Plan

Week 1

Day 1:
- Breakfast: Greek Yogurt Parfait
- Lunch: Turkey and Avocado Wrap
- Dinner: Baked Salmon with Sweet Potato and Broccoli
- Snack/Dessert: Apple Slices with Almond Butter

Day 2:
- Breakfast: Chia Seed Pudding
- Lunch: Turkey and Avocado Wrap
- Dinner: Vegetable Stir-Fry with Tofu
- Snack/Dessert: Carrot Cake Energy Bites

Day 3:
- Breakfast: Oatmeal with Berries and Almonds
- Lunch: Lentil Soup with Whole Grain Bread
- Dinner: Stuffed Bell Peppers with Ground Turkey and Brown Rice
- Snack/Dessert: Greek Yogurt with Honey and Walnuts

Day 4:
- Breakfast: Banana-Oat Cookies
- Lunch: Spinach and Artichoke Dip with Whole Grain Crackers
- Dinner: Chicken and Vegetable Skewers with Quinoa
- Snack/Dessert: Mixed Berries with Greek Yogurt

Day 5:
- Breakfast: Smoothie with Spinach, Banana, and Almond Milk
- Lunch: Chickpea Salad Sandwich on Whole Grain Bread
- Dinner: Baked Cod with Lemon and Herbs, served with Steamed Asparagus
- Snack/Dessert: Almond Butter Energy Balls

Day 6:
- Breakfast: Avocado Toast with Whole Grain Bread
- Lunch: Greek Salad with Grilled Chicken
- Dinner: Lentil and Vegetable Curry with Brown Rice
- Snack/Dessert: Cottage Cheese with Fresh Fruit

Day 7:
- Breakfast: Blueberry Pancakes made with Whole Grain Flour
- Lunch: Quinoa and Black Bean Salad
- Dinner: Grilled Salmon with Dill Sauce, served with Steamed Green Beans
- Snack/Dessert: Greek Yogurt Bark with Mixed Berries

Week 2

Day 1:
- Breakfast: Greek Yogurt Parfait
- Lunch: Quinoa Salad
- Dinner: Baked Salmon with Sweet Potato and Broccoli
- Snack/Dessert: Apple Slices with Almond Butter

Day 2:
- Breakfast: Chia Seed Pudding
- Lunch: Turkey and Avocado Wrap
- Dinner: Vegetable Stir-Fry with Tofu
- Snack/Dessert:

Day 3:
- Breakfast: Oatmeal with Berries and Almonds
- Lunch: Lentil Soup with Whole Grain Bread
- Dinner: Stuffed Bell Peppers with Ground Turkey and Brown Rice
- Snack/Dessert: Greek Yogurt with Honey and Walnuts

Day 4:
- Breakfast: Banana-Oat Cookies
- Lunch: Spinach and Artichoke Dip with Whole Grain Crackers

- Dinner: Chicken and Vegetable Skewers with Quinoa
- Snack/Dessert: Mixed Berries with Greek Yogurt

Day 5:
- Breakfast: Smoothie with Spinach, Banana, and Almond Milk
- Lunch: Chickpea Salad Sandwich on Whole Grain Bread
- Dinner: Baked Cod with Lemon and Herbs, served with Steamed Asparagus
- Snack/Dessert: Almond Butter Energy Balls

Day 6:
- Breakfast: Avocado Toast with Whole Grain Bread
- Lunch: Greek Salad with Grilled Chicken
- Dinner: Lentil and Vegetable Curry with Brown Rice
- Snack/Dessert: Cottage Cheese with Fresh Fruit

Day 7:
- Breakfast: Blueberry Pancakes made with Whole Grain Flour
- Lunch: Quinoa and Black Bean Salad
- Dinner: Baked Chicken with Rosemary and Garlic, served with Roasted Brussels Sprouts
- Snack/Dessert: Greek Yogurt Bark with Mixed Berries

Week 3

Day 1:
- Breakfast: Greek Yogurt Parfait
- Lunch: Turkey and Avocado Wrap
- Dinner: Vegetable Stir-Fry with Tofu
- Snack/Dessert: Carrot Cake Energy Bites

Day 2:
- Breakfast: Chia Seed Pudding
- Lunch: Lentil Soup with Whole Grain Bread
- Dinner: Stuffed Bell Peppers with Ground Turkey and Brown Rice

- Snack/Dessert: Greek Yogurt with Honey and Walnuts

Day 3:
- Breakfast: Oatmeal with Berries and Almonds
- Lunch: Spinach and Artichoke Dip with Whole Grain Crackers
- Dinner: Chicken and Vegetable Skewers with Quinoa
- Snack/Dessert: Mixed Berries with Greek Yogurt

Day 4:
- Breakfast: Banana-Oat Cookies
- Lunch: Greek Salad with Grilled Chicken
- Dinner: Lentil and Vegetable Curry with Brown Rice
- Snack/Dessert: Almond Butter Energy Balls

Day 5:
- Breakfast: Smoothie with Spinach, Banana, and Almond Milk
- Lunch: Chickpea Salad Sandwich on Whole Grain Bread
- Dinner: Baked Cod with Lemon and Herbs, served with Steamed Asparagus
- Snack/Dessert: Cottage Cheese with Fresh Fruit

Day 6:
- Breakfast: Avocado Toast with Whole Grain Bread
- Lunch: Quinoa and Black Bean Salad
- Dinner: Baked Chicken with Rosemary and Garlic, served with Roasted Brussels Sprouts
- Snack/Dessert: Greek Yogurt Bark with Mixed Berries

Day 7:
- Breakfast: Blueberry Pancakes made with Whole Grain Flour
- Lunch: Quinoa Salad with Roasted Vegetables
- Dinner: Grilled Salmon with Dill Sauce, served with Steamed Green Beans
- Snack/Dessert: Carrot Cake Energy Bites

Week 4

Day 1:
- Breakfast: Greek Yogurt Parfait
- Lunch: Turkey and Avocado Wrap
- Dinner: Vegetable Stir-Fry with Tofu
- Snack/Dessert: Carrot Cake Energy Bites

Day 2:
- Breakfast: Chia Seed Pudding
- Lunch: Lentil Soup with Whole Grain Bread
- Dinner: Stuffed Bell Peppers with Ground Turkey and Brown Rice
- Snack/Dessert: Greek Yogurt with Honey and Walnuts

Day 3:
- Breakfast: Oatmeal with Berries and Almonds
- Lunch: Spinach and Artichoke Dip with Whole Grain Crackers
- Dinner: Chicken and Vegetable Skewers with Quinoa
- Snack/Dessert: Mixed Berries with Greek Yogurt

Day 4:
- Breakfast: Banana-Oat Cookies
- Lunch: Greek Salad with Grilled Chicken
- Dinner: Lentil and Vegetable Curry with Brown Rice
- Snack/Dessert: Almond Butter Energy Balls

Day 5:
- Breakfast: Smoothie with Spinach, Banana, and Almond Milk
- Lunch: Chickpea Salad Sandwich on Whole Grain Bread
- Dinner: Baked Cod with Lemon and Herbs, served with Steamed Asparagus
- Snack/Dessert: Cottage Cheese with Fresh Fruit

Day 6:
- Breakfast: Avocado Toast with Whole Grain Bread

- Lunch: Quinoa and Black Bean Salad
- Dinner: Baked Chicken with Rosemary and Garlic, served with Roasted Brussels Sprouts
- Snack/Dessert: Greek Yogurt Bark with Mixed Berries

Day 7:
- Breakfast: Blueberry Pancakes made with Whole Grain Flour
- Lunch: Quinoa Salad with Roasted Vegetables
- Dinner: Grilled Salmon with Dill Sauce, served with Steamed Green Beans
- Snack/Dessert: Apple Slices with Almond Butter

Conclusion

As you embark on this journey to support your loved one with Alzheimer's through dietary changes, remember that every step you take is a step towards improving their quality of life. The Alzheimer's diet is not just about nourishing the body but also nurturing the soul and mind.

It's about creating moments of joy and connection through shared meals and shared experiences. It's about providing comfort and care through food that not only sustains the body but also nourishes the spirit.

As you prepare these meals with love and compassion, know that you are making a difference in the life of your loved one. Your dedication and commitment are truly commendable, and I hope this cookbook serves as a valuable resource and source of inspiration on your caregiving journey.

Together, we can make a difference, one meal at a time. Thank you for your love, your care, and your unwavering support.

www.ingramcontent.com/pod-product-compliance
Lightning Source LLC
Chambersburg PA
CBHW062116220526
45471CB00010B/3760